365 Days of Positive Affirmations

Pol Leon

Positive affirmation n°1: I make others around me happy.

Positive affirmation n°2: I enjoy every breath I take.

Positive affirmation n°3: I give unconditional love.

Positive affirmation n°4: I think very highly of myself because it is deserved.

Positive affirmation n°5: I am an example of confidence.

Positive affirmation n°6: I will press on and go forward.

Positive affirmation n°7: I can be soft in my heart and firm in my boundaries.

Positive affirmation n°8: I love myself.

Positive affirmation n°9: I will allow myself to evolve.

Positive affirmation n°10: I show my loved one often how much I appreciate them.

Positive affirmation n°11: My partner and I are perfectly matched.

Positive affirmation n°12: I have come farther than I would have ever thought possible, and I'm learning along the way.

Positive affirmation n°13: I see the good in all things and situations.

Positive affirmation n°14: I will always have a positive outlook and will always be optimistic.

Positive affirmation n°15: Every day I embody the best version of myself.

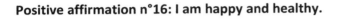

Positive affirmation n°16: I am happy and healthy.

Positive affirmation n°17: I know my worth.

Positive affirmation n°18: Nothing can stand in my way.

Positive affirmation n°19: I only speak positively.

Positive affirmation n°20: Today and every day I am blessed.

Positive affirmation n°21: My relationship is full of joy and wonder.

Positive affirmation n°22: I welcome the wisdom that comes with growing older.

Positive affirmation n°23: My soulmate is out there.

Positive affirmation n°24: It's okay to have fun.

Positive affirmation n°25: I am loved and wanted by my partner.

Positive affirmation n°26: I am beautiful and loved by everyone.

Positive affirmation n°27: I am open to healing.

Positive affirmation n°28: I make bold and smart choices.

Positive affirmation n°29: I feel okay about doing things just for me.

Positive affirmation n°30: I practice gratitude for all that I have, and all that is yet to come.

Positive affirmation n°51: My heart is open with trust.

Positive affirmation n°52: I have a fun and exciting relationship.

Positive affirmation n°53: I have everything I need inside to live a happy fulfilling life.

Positive affirmation n°54: I release all the hurt that was done to me.

Positive affirmation n°55: My life is not a race or competition.

Positive affirmation n°56: My opinions are important and they matter.

Positive affirmation n°57: The Universe is working for me.

Positive affirmation n°58: I let go of the things that sit achingly out of reach.

Positive affirmation n°59: There is strength in quiet, there is vulnerability in being loud.

Positive affirmation n°60: My relationship is stronger than any obstacle.

Positive affirmation n°81: My love is faithful and supporting.

Positive affirmation n°82: I easily overcome stress and anxiety.

Positive affirmation n°83: Great things always come my way.

Positive affirmation n°84: I have everything I need to succeed.

Positive affirmation n°85: I am worthy of investing in myself.

Positive affirmation n°86: I enjoy being in a strong, committed relationship.

Positive affirmation n°87: I constantly make positive changes in all areas of my life.

Positive affirmation n°88: I choose happiness for my life.

Positive affirmation n°89: I welcome love with open arms.

Positive affirmation n°90: The Universe is finding my perfect match.

Positive affirmation n°111: I do all things in love.

Positive affirmation n°112: My body is healthy; my mind is brilliant; my soul is tranquil.

Positive affirmation n°113: My heart knows its own way.

Positive affirmation n°114: I am energized.

Positive affirmation n°115: What matters most is how I react and what I believe.

Positive affirmation n°116: I always find the positive in everything.

Positive affirmation n°117: I am the architect of my life; I build its foundation and choose its contents.

Positive affirmation n°118: I'm doing my best and that is enough.

Positive affirmation n°119: When I feel fear, I feed trust.

Positive affirmation n°120: There is growth in stillness.

Positive affirmation n°121: My glass is always half full.

Positive affirmation n°122: Every day I appreciate myself more and more.

Positive affirmation n°123: I can control how I respond to things that are confronting.

Positive affirmation n°124: I breath in healing, I exhale the painful things that burden my heart.

Positive affirmation n°125: The greatest gift I can receive is my own unconditional love.

Positive affirmation n°126: I have the power to be happy no matter the circumstance.

Positive affirmation n°127: It's okay for me to give of myself.

Positive affirmation n°128: There is something in this world that only I can do. That is why I am here.

Positive affirmation n°129: I hold wisdom beyond knowledge.

Positive affirmation n°130: There is nothing that can come between my partner and I.

Positive affirmation n°131: I deserve to be successful and happy.

Positive affirmation n°132: I am perfect all by myself.

Positive affirmation n°133: I leave room in my life for spontaneity.

Positive affirmation n°134: I emotionally support my partner.

Positive affirmation n°135: I attract positive, loving, people in my life.

Positive affirmation n°136: I can adapt, grow, and change when necessary with ease.

Positive affirmation n°137: My feelings deserve names, deserve recognition, deserve to be felt.

Positive affirmation n°138: I confidently and respectfully speak my mind.

Positive affirmation n°139: I am my partner's rock through thick and thin.

Positive affirmation n°140: I attract love from being myself.

Positive affirmation n°141: I am blessed with amazing family and friends.

Positive affirmation n°142: I am joyful for even the simplest of things.

Positive affirmation n°143: I am an effective communicator.

Positive affirmation n°144: I alone hold the truth of who I am.

Positive affirmation n°145: I am loved and worthy.

Positive affirmation n°146: I'm worthy of respect and acceptance.

Positive affirmation n°147: I am just as good as everyone else.

Positive affirmation n°148: My life is fulfilling and full of happiness.

Positive affirmation n°149: My body is perfect in the way it's intended to be.

Positive affirmation n°150: I attract abundance into my life.

Positive affirmation n°151: I always succeed because I want to.

Positive affirmation n°152: My ability to conquer my challenges is limitless; my potential to succeed is infinite.

Positive affirmation n°153: I release all negativity.

Positive affirmation n°154: There is something in this world that only I can do. That is why I am here.

Positive affirmation n°155: Though these times are difficult, they are only a short phase of life.

Positive affirmation n°156: I see the best in myself and others.

Positive affirmation n°157: I act in all things with confidence.

Positive affirmation n°158: I am a loving and supporting husband.

Positive affirmation n°159: When I speak my needs, I receive them abundantly.

Positive affirmation n°160: Love flows towards me and through me.

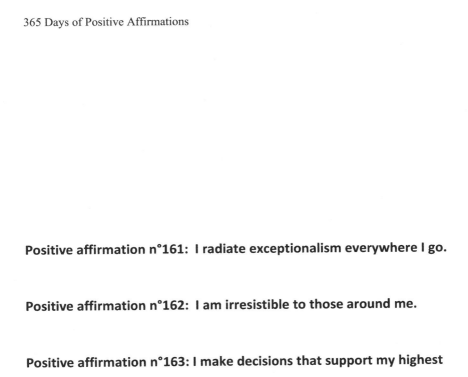

Positive affirmation n°161: I radiate exceptionalism everywhere I go.

Positive affirmation n°162: I am irresistible to those around me.

Positive affirmation n°163: I make decisions that support my highest good.

Positive affirmation n°164: I have unlimited potential. There are no limits before me.

Positive affirmation n°165: I will accomplish all my tasks today.

Positive affirmation n°166: I am the poster child for optimism.

Positive affirmation n°167: It is my birthright to live a happy and prosperous life.

Positive affirmation n°168: I am deserving of what I desire, and I will achieve it.

Positive affirmation n°169: I enjoy my spouse being so attracted to me.

Positive affirmation n°170: I am thankful for all that I have.

Positive affirmation n°171: Love surrounds me every day in every way.

Positive affirmation n°172: I wake each morning with a smile.

Positive affirmation n°173: Words may shape me, but they do not make me. I am here already.

Positive affirmation n°174: I always attract the best circumstances.

Positive affirmation n°175: I am a magnificent, radiant being.

Positive affirmation n°176: It's easy to overcome negative thoughts and emotions.

Positive affirmation n°177: Everything I need to succeed is within me.

Positive affirmation n°178: I tell the truth about who I am and what I need from others.

Positive affirmation n°179: I am superior to negative thoughts and low actions.

Positive affirmation n°180: My love is perfect inside and out.

Positive affirmation n°181: I body go after what I want in life.

Positive affirmation n°182: I have the power to change.

Positive affirmation n°183: Life is full of excitement and fun.

Positive affirmation n°184: I'm more at ease every day.

Positive affirmation n°185: I have been given endless talents which I begin to utilize today.

Positive affirmation n°186: I invite art and music into my life.

Positive affirmation n°187: Every day in every way I'm getting better and better.

Positive affirmation n°188: My confidence is unshakeable and is never diminished.

Positive affirmation n°189: I seek out mystery in the ordinary.

Positive affirmation n°190: My mind is full of positive, loving thoughts.

Positive affirmation n°191: The Universe is causing my desires to manifest.

Positive affirmation n°192: Sometimes the work is resting.

Positive affirmation n°193: I am bold and outgoing.

Positive affirmation n°194: I embrace change seamlessly and rise to the new opportunity it presents.

Positive affirmation n°195: I am complete as I am, others simply support me.

Positive affirmation n°196: I am resilient.

Positive affirmation n°197: I accept and love everything about myself.

Positive affirmation n°198: I can do anything I put my mind to.

Positive affirmation n°199: I take the time to slow down and appreciate life.

Positive affirmation n°200: There are no limits to the amount of happiness I can experience.

Positive affirmation n°201: I am an amazing wife.

Positive affirmation n°202: There is peace in changing your mind when it is done in love.

Positive affirmation n°203: I am attracting my soulmate.

Positive affirmation n°204: I'm allowed to take time to heal.

Positive affirmation n°205: I release the fears that do not serve me.

Positive affirmation n°206: I am adaptable.

Positive affirmation n°207: I am able and willing to forgive.

Positive affirmation n°208: My soul is full of love and warmth.

Positive affirmation n°209: I spread joy to everyone I meet.

Positive affirmation n°210: I'm open to new adventures in my life.

Positive affirmation n°211: My love of life spreads to others.

Positive affirmation n°212: I make time to experience grief and sadness when necessary.

Positive affirmation n°213: Happiness is a choice. I base my happiness on my own accomplishments and the blessings I've been given.

Positive affirmation n°214: I am grateful for everything I have been blessed with.

Positive affirmation n°215: I am beautiful inside and out.

Positive affirmation n°216: I love who I am.

Positive affirmation n°217: I hold community for others, and am held in community by others.

Positive affirmation n°218: Saying no is an act of self-affirmation, too.

Positive affirmation n°219: I smile at everyone I walk by.

Positive affirmation n°220: I clearly see all opportunities in front of me.

Positive affirmation n°221: I can be me in my relationship.

Positive affirmation n°222: I am living an excellent life.

Positive affirmation n°223: The Universe is delivering freedom and happiness.

Positive affirmation n°224: The power to be happy relies in only me.

Positive affirmation n°225: Difficult times allow me to appreciate the good times.

Positive affirmation n°226: My choices are wise and sound.

Positive affirmation n°227: I grow towards my interests, like a plant reaching for the sun.

Positive affirmation n°228: I create a positive atmosphere everywhere I go.

Positive affirmation n°229: I choose to think of myself and others in a positive light.

Positive affirmation n°230: I am confident in my love life.

Positive affirmation n°231: I am responsible for myself, and I start there.

Positive affirmation n°232: I am a victor not a victim.

Positive affirmation n°233: I have a positive outlook no matter the situation.

Positive affirmation n°234: I am meeting my soulmate today.

Positive affirmation n°235: I am valued and helpful.

Positive affirmation n°236: I make time for things that make me happy.

Positive affirmation n°237: I am superior to negative thoughts.

Positive affirmation n°238: My perspective is unique and important.

Positive affirmation n°239: I easily accept compliments because I deserve them.

Positive affirmation n°240: I'm in control of how I react to others.

Positive affirmation n°241: I uplift my joy and the joy of others.

Positive affirmation n°242: There is room for me at the table.

Positive affirmation n°243: I know that happiness comes from great habits.

Positive affirmation n°244: I am capable of overcoming anything.

Positive affirmation n°245: I deserve to feel joy.

Positive affirmation n°246: I easily create habits that are healthy for me.

Positive affirmation n°247: I love to have fun.

Positive affirmation n°248: Peace is my middle name.

Positive affirmation n°249: Fear of failure does not control me.

Positive affirmation n°250: I am easily conquering my sickness.

Positive affirmation n°251: I belong here, and I deserve to take up space.

Positive affirmation n°252: I will succeed today.

Positive affirmation n°253: I learn and grow through difficulty.

Positive affirmation n°254: I feed my body and mind with positive thoughts.

Positive affirmation n°255: I have everything I need to succeed.

Positive affirmation n°256: Every day my spouse and I strengthen our bond.

Positive affirmation n°257: My goal is to listen and understand, not to win.

Positive affirmation n°258: I love being alive.

Positive affirmation n°259: I always overcome obstacles.

Positive affirmation n°260: I realize that everything that happens is for a reason.

Positive affirmation n°261: I am attracting the right love.

Positive affirmation n°262: My spouse and I are meant to be together.

Positive affirmation n°263: Happiness exists everywhere I go.

Positive affirmation n°264: I am capable of balancing ease and effort in my life.

Positive affirmation n°265: I am completely whole and happy by myself.

Positive affirmation n°266: I embrace failure and learn from it.

Positive affirmation n°267: I am on my game.

Positive affirmation n°268: I wake up in a positive mood.

Positive affirmation n°269: I am still learning so it's okay to make mistakes.

Positive affirmation n°270: I am courageous and I stand up for myself.

Positive affirmation n°271: My past is not a reflection of my future.

Positive affirmation n°272: My body is powerful.

Positive affirmation n°273: Thinking positive is a natural part of who I am.

Positive affirmation n°274: My thoughts are filled with positivity.

Positive affirmation n°275: I respect myself highly.

Positive affirmation n°276: I'm going to have a great day.

Positive affirmation n°277: My thoughts are filled with positivity and my life is plentiful with prosperity.

Positive affirmation n°278: I am surrounded by people who love and support me.

Positive affirmation n°279: Every decision I make is supported by my whole and inarguable experience.

Positive affirmation n°280: I take the time to be mindful of my surroundings.

Positive affirmation n°281: My life gets better as I get older.

Positive affirmation n°282: I will see today's work through.

Positive affirmation n°283: I deserve self-respect and a clean space.

Positive affirmation n°284: I look forward to tomorrow and the opportunities that await me.

Positive affirmation n°285: I support myself fully and competently.

Positive affirmation n°286: Joy comes easy for me.

Positive affirmation n°287: I can hold two opposing feelings at once, it means I am processing.

Positive affirmation n°288: I am brimming with great ideas.

Positive affirmation n°289: Today I celebrate that I am younger than I'm ever going to be.

Positive affirmation n°290: I am optimistic because today is a new day.

Positive affirmation n°291: My positivity transforms my reality.

Positive affirmation n°292: I love every aspect of my life.

Positive affirmation n°293: I am responsible for my happiness, no one else is.

Positive affirmation n°294: I can get through hardship.

Positive affirmation n°295: Confidence allows me to overcome procrastination and take action.

Positive affirmation n°296: I choose not to criticize myself or others around me.

Positive affirmation n°297: Asking for help is a sign of self-respect and self-awareness.

Positive affirmation n°298: I will heal from this.

Positive affirmation n°299: I am powerful.

Positive affirmation n°300: The love I give is increased many times when it comes back to me.

Positive affirmation n°301: I can hold two opposing feelings at once, it means I am processing.

Positive affirmation n°302: I am positive.

Positive affirmation n°303: I know exactly what to do to achieve success.

Positive affirmation n°304: My high self-esteem allows me to shrug off criticism easily.

Positive affirmation n°305: Gaining strength and wisdom from failure comes naturally.

Positive affirmation n°306: I do not have to linger in dark places; there is help for me here.

Positive affirmation n°307: I trust the person I am becoming.

Positive affirmation n°308: I am courageous.

Positive affirmation n°309: I am in a joyous, fulfilling relationship with a person who loves me more than anything.

Positive affirmation n°310: I forgive those who have hurt me.

Positive affirmation n°311: I release the past.

Positive affirmation n°312: I have unbreakable confidence.

Positive affirmation n°313: I appreciate who I am and love my life.

Positive affirmation n°314: I welcome the wisdom that comes with growing older.

Positive affirmation n°315: I let go of all that no longer serves me.

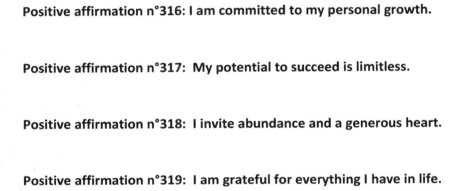

Positive affirmation n°316: I am committed to my personal growth.

Positive affirmation n°317: My potential to succeed is limitless.

Positive affirmation n°318: I invite abundance and a generous heart.

Positive affirmation n°319: I am grateful for everything I have in life.

Positive affirmation n°320: I welcome into my life an abundance of joy.

Positive affirmation n°321: I am in love with being in love.

Positive affirmation n°322: I breathe in trust, I exhale doubt.

Positive affirmation n°323: I choose to be happy.

Positive affirmation n°324: I am deserving of love just the way I am.

Positive affirmation n°325: My body is beautiful in this moment and at its current size.

Positive affirmation n°326: I am well rested.

Positive affirmation n°327: I deserve to feel good about myself.

Positive affirmation n°328: I go for what I want without hesitation.

Positive affirmation n°329: I can do anything I want.

Positive affirmation n°330: When I talk to myself as I would a friend, I see all my best qualities and I allow myself to shine.

Positive affirmation n°331: I release what no longer serves me.

Positive affirmation n°332: I am well-rested and excited for the day.

Positive affirmation n°333: I am creative, talented, and confident.

Positive affirmation n°334: Today, I am brimming with energy and overflowing with joy.

Positive affirmation n°335: I attract peace and love.

Positive affirmation n°336: I always act in the face of fear.

Positive affirmation n°337: I am proof enough of who I am and what I deserve.

Positive affirmation n°338: I understand that every moment I breathe is a gift.

Positive affirmation n°339: I celebrate the good qualities in others and myself.

Positive affirmation n°340: My actions are for my future, not because of my past.

Positive affirmation n°341: I easily make friends.

Positive affirmation n°342: I am naturally confident in all that I do.

Positive affirmation n°343: I am wise and humble.

Positive affirmation n°344: I am strong enough to make my own decisions.

Positive affirmation n°345: My partner knows me and loves me flaws and all.

Positive affirmation n°346: I am held and supported by those who love me.

Positive affirmation n°347: My inner beauty is shining through.

Positive affirmation n°348: All is well.

Positive affirmation n°349: Letting go creates space for opportunities to come.

Positive affirmation n°350: I am attractive, I am beautiful, I am desirable.

Positive affirmation n°351: I can do anything I put my mind to.

Positive affirmation n°352: I create love all around me.

Positive affirmation n°353: There is poetry in everything, if I look for it.

Positive affirmation n°354: To make small steps toward big goals is progress.

Positive affirmation n°355: When I release shame, I move into myself more beautifully.

Positive affirmation n°356: I believe in myself.

Positive affirmation n°357: I can create my own true happiness.

Positive affirmation n°358: I empty my mind of all negative thoughts.

Positive affirmation n°359: My mind is clear.

Positive affirmation n°360: I act swiftly and with energy.

Positive affirmation n°361: I'm in charge of my life and no one will dictate my path besides me.

Positive affirmation n°362: Many people look up to me and recognize my worth; I am admired.

Positive affirmation n°363: I am joyous about my opportunities.

Positive affirmation n°364: I speak kind, supporting words to my partner.

Positive affirmation n°365: My needs and wants are important.

Made in the USA
Middletown, DE
24 September 2022